Table of Contents

WRITTEN DOCUMENTS YOU SHOULD HAVE

Living will

Before you enter a nursing home make sure you have a Living Will. A Living Will details a person's desires regarding their medical treatment when they are not able to give informed consent (advance directive).

Written will

You should have a written will. A simple will could be a written statement of how you want your assets to be transferred after your death. If you don't have a will when you die, the state you live in could decide how your property should be distributed.

Durable power of attorney for finances

You should have a durable power of attorney for finances. The person you choose would have the authority to do specific things for you, such as signing your checks, pay your bills or sell property for you. If a power of attorney is durable, that means it remains in effect if you should become unable to make decisions for yourself. If a power of attorney is not durable, it ends if you become unable to make your own decisions.

Durable power of attorney for health care

You will also need a durable power of attorney for health care. This allows someone to make medical decisions for you if you are not able to speak for yourself. If you do not have these documents a social worker at the nursing home should be able to help you fill them out or find someone to come in and help you fill them out.

Sit down with the person you would like to be your durable power of attorney for finances and your durable power of attorney for health care and make sure they understand what you want done. The day you break a hip is not the day to have that discussion. Check on the internet to see what your state requires to appoint someone your power of attorney and how to make a living will. For example if you go to: http://www.dhs.wisconsin.gov/forms/advdirectives/ F00085.pdf you can get the living will form and instructions on how to fill it out that's accepted in Wisconsin (advanced directives would be a living will). If you do not feel comfortable doing these forms on your own, your attorney should be able to help you fill them out or, as I stated previously, the nursing home social worker should be able to help you. Another option would be to check with any agency on aging in your area.

The Federal Citizen Information Center created the free Family Caregivers Kit. Publications from the Consumer Financial Protection Bureau explain how to manage a loved one's money and protect seniors from scams. It also contains publications from the FDA's Office of Women's Health to keep track of medications and learn to use them safely. The kit has tips that helps caregivers manage a loved one's affairs.

http://www.medicare.gov/campaigns/caregiver/caregiver.html

PAYING FOR YOUR HEALTH CARE

Insurance/Medicare/Medicaid coverage is confusing. Ask specific questions when you are trying to find out what is covered and how much you will have to pay out-of-pocket.

Medicare A and Medicare A replacement

Many people get the impression that Medicare and some Medicare replacement insurances automatically cover your nursing home stay if you have had a qualifying hospital stay. You would have to be receiving skilled nursing or therapy services for this to be true. If you reach a point where you no longer need those services, you would no longer be eligible for Medicare A coverage. Medicare does not always provide 100% of coverage for the full 100 days that can be allowed.
For more information on Medicare A go to:
http://www.medicare.gov/what-medicarecovers/part-a/w

Medicare B and Medicare B replacement

Medicare B is coverage for preventative services and medically necessary services and supplies to treat or diagnose your medical condition. That would include lab tests, doctor visits, wheelchairs and walkers. You generally pay 20% of the Medicare-approved amount for the doctor or other health care provider's services, and the Part B deductible applies.
For more information on Medicare go to:
http://www.medicare.gov/Pubs/pdf/10116.pdf

Medicaid

Medicaid policy also confuses people. Medicaid is a Federal-State health insurance program for low income and needy people, which covers children, the aged, blind, and/or disabled and other people who are eligible to receive federally assisted income maintenance payments.
When anyone over 55, who is a Medicare recipient dies, all states are required to recover the expense of long-term care and related costs. States also have the option to recover all other Medicaid expenses. Do not think you will be living in a nursing home on Medicaid's dollar and be able to leave all your property to anyone.
Living at home on Medicaid is a whole different kettle of fish than living in a long term care facility so get some good advice before you decide to sell any property and consult an elder law attorney.

Here are good sites to get some answers:
https://www.caring.com/questions/pay-
backmedicaid-after-selling-house
http://www.consumerreports.org/cro/news/2014/0
1/will-medicaid-take-my-house-when-i-
die/index.htm http://www.elderlawanswers.com/

Veterans

Veterans who are living in long term care facilities
other than those provided by the Veterans
Administration can still go to VA doctors for
treatment. Don't forget to check with your local
Veterans Administration about what drugs you can
receive through the VA This site gives a guide about
paying for long term care :
http://www.va.gov/geriatrics/guide/longtermcare/
P aying_for_Long_Term_Care.asp
This site is an interactive map to help you find
facilities in each state:
http://www.va.gov/directory/guide/home.asp?isfla
s h=1

[Don't wait until you need to use your insurance to
find out what it will cover. Read the insurance
coverage booklet and ask questions. Make the
questions specific, 'What happens if I break my hip
and have to go to a nursing home? Will I be covered
100%? How long will I have complete coverage?
When and why would the coverage end? What if my
skilled services come to an end but I don't think I'm
ready to go home yet?']

BEFORE YOU DECIDE-
VISIT

Staff to resident ratio

What's the staff to resident ratio? Find out what the number of residents to nursing assistants and the number of residents to nurses is. This can have a huge impact on quality of care. This can range from 1:5 up to 1:20 for CNAs and 1:20 to 1:80 for nursing staff. (Note: A certified nursing assistant, or CNA, helps patients or clients with healthcare needs under the supervision of a Registered Nurse (RN) or a Licensed Practical Nurse (LPN).

What does the nursing home look like and smell like over-all?

If you smell poop when you visit, walk back through 45 minutes later--if you STILL smell poop, there's a problem. Is the staff friendly or do they appear to be hurried? **Go during an evening meal** and see what the meals are like. Do you have choices for your meals? Do you have to eat at a set time or can you decide when to eat? Is there enough staff to help everyone who needs help eating and drinking? Is the staff focused on the person they are helping or are they chatting among themselves? Are they taking people right from the dining area and putting them to bed? I said to go for an evening meal because the nursing home staff will expect visitors during daytime hours and weekends, not so much during the week, toward evening. During the daytime hours there are more administrators and social workers etc. around watching how things are done. Are we trying to catch them doing something wrong? No, we are trying to catch them doing the right thing.

A **call light** is fastened to the wall in a room, that when turned on signals the nursing station, indicating that the patient has a need requiring attention from the CNA on duty. Usually these are attached to a light outside the resident's room that will come on when activated. Keep an eye on these lights when you are visiting. Are there a lot of unanswered lights on with CNAs standing or sitting in a group talking? How long is it before they are answered?

Will you have any input on **potential roommates**? Would you like someone who likes to visit or someone quiet? Will your television bother her or hers bother you? If you are of sound mind will it bother you to have a roommate with dementia? Where will your room be located? If it's at the end of the hall, it could be quiet but also make it more difficult to get to activities or the dining room. How much help do you require getting around? If you are still mobile, whether walking or in a wheelchair, it could be good exercise for you to travel a long hallway. If you have health issues that would make the journey difficult it may be a good idea to ask if a closer room is available.

Is the room attractive with nice curtains and comforter? Does it look institutionalized? If you like the nursing home but are put off by the room consider asking about adding your own touches such as pictures, your own comforter and curtains or valence.

Staff interaction with residents

How does the staff interact with the residents? Are the people living there treated with respect and as adults? I would not like someone to talk 'baby talk' to me, treat me like a child or talk as if I'm not in the room no matter how much dementia I may have. Some people feel very strongly about being called by their married name, 'Mrs. Jones' for example. The staff should be speaking to the residents in a respectful way and engage each person one-on-one.

The Room

Making the room your own can be a challenge. Being in a nursing home doesn't mean you cannot have any of your things from your previous residence. Talk to the administrator and find out how big your room will be. Some nursing homes have **private rooms available for an extra cost**. Many people live in a room with one other person and share a bathroom. Sometimes you can fit in a favorite chair (vinyl or leather if possible), there is always wall space for your photos and usually a small amount of dresser top space where you might want to put a plant. Trying to bring too much can be overwhelming for you and a possible roommate. It's time to make tough decisions on what to get rid of and what you can take.

Do you have a favorite blanket or pillow? There should be no reason you can't have that on your bed. In fact, if your bed will fit, you may be able to have it moved in. Don't forget about a **television, radio or computer**. A wall mount for your television might be a good idea or a laptop instead of a desktop computer. A tablet reader would be a good idea so you don't have to worry about running out of reading material if you like to read.

[Remember that you will probably be responsible for any internet connection, television connection or phone connection you decide you want to have.]

For the **safety** of all residents and staff, the nursing home must check any equipment, furniture and electrical appliances that you wish to bring. Before you plug in your own television, computer or fan the nursing home will want to inspect any cords to make sure they are not frayed and everything is in good working condition and up to fire code. You will not be able to use extension cords because that could be a trip hazard.

Is there a mirror you can actually see yourself in and a closet with a lower rod that you can reach if you are in a wheelchair? Is the nursing home willing to make those changes if need be?

Don't forget, you can **decorate your room for the holidays** too. Enlist the help of friends and family to help hang decorations or set up a table top tree. Some homes have a limited amount of **storage space** that you can use to store out of season clothes and a few personal items like this. Otherwise your family may have to store them. The Activity Department often can contribute decorations and help put them up.

For more information on choosing a nursing home go to this site:

http://www.medicare.gov/pubs/pdf/02174.pdf

So I've moved in. Now what?

You have decided this is the nursing home for you. What's next?

CALL LIGHT

One of the most important things to check is the call light. A call light is a gadget you should be able to press/pull to alert the nursing assistants (CNA) that you need help. **There should be two call lights, one by your bed and one in the bathroom. Make sure they are where you can reach them.** Often the one by the bed is clipped to the top bed cover or wrapped around the short side rail on the bed. If you push it, it should turn on the light above your bed and a light outside your door. If it isn't answered and turned off in a matter of minutes, an alert should sound at the nurses' station (located as a central hub at the end of the hallways).

The call light in the bathroom is usually next to the stool with a string you pull down. If you are not able to grip a string or push the button to turn the call light on, there are **options of pads that you tap with your hand**. You should never have to wait 15 minutes for your light to be answered. If you find this is happening (be sure to time it with a clock/watch because 5 minutes can seem like 15 if you have to use the toilet), make sure the call light is working correctly (sometimes they aren't firmly plugged in or just plain fail).

If it is working and is still not getting answered keep a log of the time of day, the CNA, the circumstance and the total time taken. Don't forget, we are all human and CNAs can get busy or unavailable for some other reason.

If a CNA makes a habit of coming in and shutting off your light with a promise to return, and doesn't, keep track of that also. OK, so you have your log, now what? Ask to talk to your social worker. (Who's that you ask?? When you were admitted to the nursing home a social worker should have been involved and that person should have regular meeting with you to see how your stay is going. This person can also take your case to the charge nurse for your wing.) If talking to your social worker doesn't seem to work or you feel your complaints are being blown off, enlist help. Have someone close to you (child, spouse, power of attorney etc.) come at the times you are experiencing the most problems (If they can slip in without being seen so much the better). Put on your call light and have them witness the time and take it to the administrator of the nursing home. Yes, go over some heads and step on some toes. Unfortunately, the squeaky wheel gets oiled.

Low Vision

Low vision is a permanent loss of vision that can be caused by glaucoma, diabetes and macular degeneration. Low vision increases the risk of falling, makes it difficult to read, recognize faces or the edges of a things (steps, bed, plate). Better lighting, contrasting colors, magnifiers and talking devices can all help you remain independent. Make sure there are clear walkways and even and adequate light levels. Use a goose neck lamp so you can direct the light where you need it. Control glare by closing drapes or blinds and don't have polished surfaces. Use large print on everything from reading material, playing cards and telephone key pads. Use Velcro or rubber bands to provide tactile cues. Talking devices can include watches and telephones. An illuminated magnifying glass or electronic magnifier can help to view pictures or print. Your name in a bright color, in large print, outside your room can help you locate your room. Plates and cups with rims and a colored band around the edge can make meals easier. A brightly colored bedspread can help distinguish the bed from the floor. Colored tape can be added to the edges of furniture.

Go to these sites for more ideas:

http://www.independentliving.com

http://www.afb.org/info/low-vision/living-with-lowvision

https://lifecenter.ric.org

GOING OUT

If you would like to go out with family, it often isn't a problem. After all it's not a 'prison' but a 'home'.   If you are independent and your own person (legally able to make your own decisions) **the nursing home would like to know if you are leaving for a meal or a day or even overnight**. They need to know something bad hasn't happened to you, to make sure you have any medications you need and that they don't make a meal you are not going to be there to eat.

 If you are not your own person, your legal guardian would have to make the decision if it's all right for you to go out.

 I did mention that sometimes you may be able to stay out overnight. This is a bit more complicated because insurance issues can play into the decision. If you want an overnight stay, I would enlist the help of your social worker.

VISITORS

Visitors can be nice or sometimes not a nice thing. If you want visitors and they call before they come, you might want to suggest **'best visiting times'**. If you are going to be out of your room having therapy or a therapist has made plans to come to your room at a specific time try to schedule your visitors around that time. If you cannot see your visitors at a different times usually therapy will work around your schedule. Most nursing homes allow visitors to buy a meal if you'd like to visit during lunch or dinner. If it's on your diet, visitors can bring in a take-out meal (more on this later). If you are eating together, ask where a good place to eat would be if you want some privacy or a more homey atmosphere.
If you like **children** and would like to spend time with them, encourage family/friends to bring their children. Often people hesitate to bring children for fear they'll make you 'nervous' or be too rowdy. Most children are fine visiting and have a good time as long as they have something to keep them busy.
 If you don't feel well and **would rather not have company**, let your nurse know so they can request visitors not to intrude. Sometimes a sign outside your door that asks visitors to check at the nursing station first is a good idea.

If you have a hard time recalling who all has visited, a **visitor book** is nice. If you have a hard time recalling when someone plans to visit, a **calendar** with that information written in is nice. A calendar with birthdays, appointments and special occasions is nice to have anyway. Ask that all your appointments be written on your calendar if you aren't able to do that yourself. Ask someone close that knows birthdays etc. to write those in if you aren't able.

PETS

Pets become a big part of our lives, members of our family. If you had to leave your pet behind but would like visits from him/her ask how that can happen. Most nursing homes allow animals to visit. If you would like your pet or family/friends would like to bring their pets to visit, all pets will have to show a certificate of **up to date vaccines**. Cats are usually crated and dogs on a leash. If the pet is not well behaved or aggressive it should not visit you in the home but you may be able to go outside to visit with him/her. Make sure the pet is **toileted** before coming into the nursing home. Potty accidents happen, so be prepared to clean up quickly, so people accidents don't happen. **Don't allow your/their pet to go up to other residents without permission.** Not everyone likes animals and some may have had a bad experience. Let's not forget allergies either.

PERSONAL APPEARANCE AND HYGIENE

Clothes

What you wear can be an evolving thing. When you first arrive at the nursing home you will probably bring what you have been wearing. The same slacks, tops, dresses, undergarments, socks and shoes will all be in your closet and dresser drawers. As time goes on you may find some of these articles of clothing no longer work for you. Can you get your pants on without feeling like you are stuffing sausage? Do the buttons on your shirt meet in the middle like they should? Often times as we age clothes are not the priority they use to be and we don't get rid of things we should. You may find that you've gained weight or lost weight. You may find that you can't do buttons anymore. You may find those zippers hard to navigate. You may find you are slipping and tripping. If you are a man and having problems keeping pants up, try suspenders. If you are able, go through your clothes and **get rid of the ones that are too tight or too big or just uncomfortable**. If you are not able to do this for yourself a caregiver should do it for you. There are also **gadgets that can help make dressing easier** if you are having problems with button, zippers or reaching (more on this later). Get rid of those sloppy, tread wore shoes **and get a good sturdy shoe with good soles.**

[Make sure all your clothing and belongings are marked with your name.]

Check once in a while to make sure articles of clothing haven't gone missing and if you see mom wearing something you don't recognize check to see if there is an identification tag inside, to make sure it's hers. If you see someone wearing clothing (or other things like watches or jewelry) that you suspect belongs to you or your loved one, ask the CNA to check for you.

Ask your dentist to mark your dentures. Even glasses and hearing aids can be engraved with a name.or initials

Take pictures and write down serial numbers of any larger items such as televisions or phones. Take pictures of the room showing the furnishings you have.

This site gives good ideas and information on how to protect your things at a long term care facility:

https://www.colorado.gov/pacific/sites/default/fil es/

HF Protecting-Personal-Property-in-a-Colorado-Nursing-Home-or-Assisted-Living-Facility.pdf

Hair, makeup and razors

Take a look at your hair. Is it a style that's easy to maintain? I'm not saying you should get a short curly perm but if you are use to an elaborate hair style, it may be difficult to keep looking good. Many nursing home have a beauty shop on site so you can get a cut and perm. Be aware that it is not free. This might be a good place for family to put Christmas or birthday cash gifts. CNAs try hard to keep you looking good and should roll up your hair after a shower. Don't get a haircut or hair style just for the sake of convenience. If you look in the mirror and don't like what you see, it can be darn depressing.

Do you wear makeup? Continue to do so. If it's hard to get that lip stick on ask the CNA to do it when you get up and dressed. You will feel more in control of your life if you continue to do things that are important to you and make you feel better about yourself. Ladies, don't be afraid to ask your CNA to pull those long, wayward chin hairs if the CNA doesn't routinely do that for you. Gentlemen, ask to get those nose hairs and bushy eyebrows trimmed. The nursing home will probably require that you use an electric razor for the safety of yourself and other residents.

Shower or bath

How often is it important to you to take a shower or bath? Most nursing homes have a once a week schedule. Some nursing homes have a whirlpool tub. If you prefer one over the other be sure to ask. If you feel like you need more than one shower/bath a week, ask. Some people are comfortable with just a good wash in between. If you like certain soaps or lotions have family bring them in. If you are allergic to certain things be sure the nursing home knows. [This is probably a good place to let you women know if you need help with your cares and you are not comfortable with a male CNA (or a man with a female CNA) let the nursing staff know. Most CNAs are wonderful, caring people who will totally understand if you have a preference.]

ROOMMATES

Unless you are able to afford to have a private room, expect to have a roommate. This means not only **shared space but shared bathroom and shared noise**. Some people like having a roommate because they like having the company and someone to share their day with. Other people have a harder time dealing with someone in their immediate area all the time. If you are the latter you may find it easier if you try to get out of your room as much as possible. Most nursing homes have alcoves or visiting areas available. You can also pull the privacy curtain for a smidge more privacy. If your roommate can't or won't understand the boundaries and it becomes a problem, talk to you social worker.
Sometimes rooms can be changed.

[If your roommate has a lot of company and it's too much for you, ask the nurse to request they go to one of the visiting areas. Having the nurse do the asking can deflect hard feelings away from you and help prevent tension between you and your roommate. This is a two way street though. If you have a lot of company, watch television or listen to the radio be considerate of your roommate.] Another issue can come up if you are short and your roommate is taller (or vice versa). A major problem can be the toilet. If you or your roommate break a hip, often the doctor will request a higher toilet seat. If one of you is 4' 10" and the other is 5' 8" and a device is added to raise the toilet seat the petite person is going to have a challenge. Most people don't like to make waves but sometimes little things can add up and make for an inconvenient, unsafe or unhappy life. If things really become a problem or make you very unhappy, it's time to talk to someone in charge.

If you are married, you and your spouse can share a room. This can be a good thing or a bad thing depending on your relationship. If you request to room with someone else, or each to have a private room, be prepared for questions about it from your children, family or other people. Sometimes a simple answer is best, like "He/she snores so much I can't sleep." It's really no one's business but yours.

DIET

The dietitian in charge of the nursing home kitchen should consult with you about the diet you want/need when you first arrive. The dietitian should be aware of any doctor orders for any dietary restrictions or special diets. **If you are your own person, you have the final say in what you will eat.** I'm sure the doctor and/or the dietitian will reiterate reasons for a certain diet if you choose not to follow it but the choice is yours.

If you are considered incompetent, your health care power of attorney will make the decision for you. If you are the HPOA don't just go with the flow. Check to see how the new diet is going. If the person you are responsible for refuses to eat because he/she doesn't like it, you may decide to let him/her eat what they want. If he or she is coughing and choking on what they want but will still eat the special ordered diet, you may decide that the diet is needed. Sometimes you may decide to stray a little from the ordered diet for a special treat. Remember quality of life should be at the top of the list.

Family and friends can bring food in for you but it would be a good idea to call your charge nurse to see if you have any restrictions before bringing it, unless you (as your own person) requested it. This would include candy, specialty foods and take-out food that you might have a craving for. If you love a snack during the day or evening, let the dietitian know. There should be several options to choose from. Many nursing homes have vending machines available where you can buy a soda pop or candy bar.

Alcoholic beverages

Alcoholic beverages are not necessarily off limits just because you are in a nursing home. Strange as it may sound, you can have your doctor write an order stating that you can continue to have an alcoholic beverage every day, either in your room or as part of a 'happy hour' set up by the activity department. So if you enjoy a glass of wine with your evening meal, chances are, you can continue to do so. You will be required to purchase your own beverage.

Doctors, Nurses, CNAs, Medical Records

Doctors

Every nursing home should have a Medical Director who is responsible for resident care policies and coordinating the medical care in the facility. Usually the Medical Director is a physician who sees residents at the nursing home also. Depending on the size of the nursing home, there should be more than one physician who comes to the nursing home to see patients on a regular basis. If you are able to go out to the clinic you have always used, you can continue to do so. The nursing home staff should help you arrange transportation if you need it. If you prefer, you can change your care over to one of the regular doctors who come into the nursing home. I would recommend finding out who they are and ask others if they have had any experiences with any of them before making a choice.

Nurses

The nursing staff may be split between charge nurses and medication nurses. A **charge nurse** is usually in charge of a specific area of the home. That nurse should be following your care and be in close contact with the CNAs who help you with your daily routine. The charge nurse is usually in direct communication with your doctor and often your family. Usually a CNA will report to the charge nurse any changes they might have noticed about your health, cognition or mental health. If you feel you have an urgent need that you want addressed, asking to see the charge nurse is often helpful. A **medication nurse** is a nurse who keeps track of and dispenses medications to you. Don't be afraid to ask what the medications are for if you get something you don't recognize. Don't be afraid to tell the medication nurse if you feel something isn't working for you. Always tell the nurse if a medication is making you dizzy, constipated or have diarrhea, blurry vision, drowsy, rash, dry mouth, or nausea.

Certified Nursing Assistants (CNA)

Certified Nursing Assistants (CNA) work under the supervision of a nurse giving care to the residents. CNAs usually help with basic care such as bathing, dressing, toileting, eating and oral care. Your CNA will come to know you better than just about anyone else and you will learn a lot about him or her. The CNAs should make sure you are cleaned up every day, your teeth are brushed after meals (esp. at night) and your hair is neat and clean. Depending on the location of the long term care facility and the facility policies, CNAs may be expected to trim nails. Long or infected toenails can be a huge danger for a diabetic person. If the resident is diabetic a podiatrist would probably do any toenail trimming. No matter who trims finger and toenails, the CNA should be aware of nails that are getting to long or fungal and report it to the nurse in charge.   While the CNAs are helping you with your cares they should be carefully looking for any areas of concern. Any red areas, bruises, cuts, abrasions, foot problems or signs of increased pain or discomfort should be reported to nursing immediately. [If you are able to get up and use the toilet, do so. This will help you void better and help prevent urinary tract infections. CNAs should not encourage you to use a bedpan for convenience. Some people find that if they have bladder urgency having a toileting schedule helps. The CNA would help you to use the toilet at a specific time, even if you feel like you don't have to use it that much. This helps head off the feeling of urgency.]

Medical Record

Your Medical Record should be at the main nurses'
station. This record should be available for you or
your HPOA to look at and the nurses or your doctor
should be willing to answer any questions you have.
Your medical record should not be out for any
unauthorized person to see and your medical
information should be shared with only those you
authorized. If you have a concern about who will see
your information let the social worker or charge nurse
know. You can also ask them, who specifically, can
see your medical record. Just because someone is a
close relative (child, sibling etc.) doesn't mean the
nursing home can give out information to that person.
If the person isn't on a signed authorization form, the
nursing home can only give out generic information,
it doesn't matter if it's your mother.

[If you are going from the nursing home to the
hospital or from one medical facility to another ask if
your medical records have been sent, including a list
of your medications. Sometimes it gets overlooked in
the shuffle and can cause a long wait as you try to get
things straightened out.]

Activity Department

Check out the Activity Department. Someone from the department should be in to visit with you shortly after you take up residence. Their job is to find out more about you; your likes and dislikes, if you like to go out and be social or stay in your room and read. After they get to know you, they should give you a list of what the department does and what is available. A good activity department should have activities for all different levels of interaction. There should be books and magazines, music and groups coming in to make music, games, cooking, men's groups, women's groups, church, outdoor activities, pet therapy, and on and on. A calendar with upcoming events on it should be left in your room. If there is an event you want to participate in, either someone from activities or a CNA should make sure you make it to it.

Some Activity Departments work with Pet Therapy animals. Usually these are certified therapy animals that make regular visits. Most facilities have rules to ensure that the animals are clean, vaccinated, well trained and screened.

Want to know more on why Activity Departments are important? Go to this site:

http://www.ltlmagazine.com/blogs/ebarbera/psychological-importance-nursing-home-activities

Therapy Departments

SPEECH AND LANGUAGE THERAPY

If you find you are having problems with some food, choking or coughing when eating or drinking, if you have problems with your speech or memory, then a visit with speech-language pathology may benefit you. SLPs work with people who have swallowing disorders and can help adults speak clearer and louder. They may be able to help with memory, attention, problem solving and strategies to compensate for impaired memory.

If you have had **multiple pneumonias**, it may be worthwhile to have a speech therapist look at your medical records and do an evaluation of your eating. Aspiration pneumonia happens when food, saliva or vomit is breathed into the lungs or airways. [CNAs should not put you back into bed immediately after eating. Lying down after a meal, can relax the ring muscle at the base of the esophagus & allow acid to reflux up the esophagus, sometimes into the mouth & throat. Refluxed food can also be aspirated into the lungs leading to aspiration pneumonia.]

Signs that you may need a swallow evaluation could include one or more of the following: cough/wheezing that becomes worse, coughing up food, heartburn, nausea and sour taste in the mouth. You may have problems swallowing with any eating or drinking, or only with certain types of foods or liquids. Difficulty eating very hot or cold foods, dry crackers or bread, meat, or chicken may be an early sign of swallowing problems.

Things that may cause a swallow problem are: certain medicines,   a brain or nerve disorder (stroke, Parkinson's, spinal cord injury, MS etc.), esophageal spasm (The muscles of the esophagus suddenly squeeze.), something is blocking your throat or esophagus, dry mouth.

Sources:

https://www.healthtap.com/user_questions
http://www.webmd.com/digestivedisorders/tc/diff iculty-swallowing-dysphagiaoverview

OCCUPATIONAL THERAPY

An occupational therapist provides therapy to all ages including older adults with physical and cognitive changes. **They help older adults to set goals and safely do the things they want to do.** If you are recovering from an illness or injury, or have a disability, occupational therapy works with you to make sure you can do all the things that are important to you. Sometimes they help you do something in a different way, sometimes they work with you to do strengthening exercises and sometimes they suggest aids to help you be as independent as possible. They will also work with the CNAs, showing them how to best help you stay as independent and as safe as possible. One of the main emphasis of occupational therapy is working with you doing your activities of daily living (ADLs).

Occupational therapy may recommend adaptive tools or work on wheelchair positioning and wheelchair cushions. OTs will often work on safe strategies for dressing or using the toilet. Occupational therapists may also focus on upper body problems such as hand pain or shoulder mobility. Often occupational therapy will include exercises and the therapist will ask you to continue them after you are discharged from therapy. See more at: http://www.aota.org/AboutOccupational-Therapy/PatientsClients/DisabilityAndRehabilitation

PHYSICAL THERAPY

Physical therapists help people improve their movement and manage their pain through the use of exercises and equipment. A physical therapist will often see elderly patients for pain, post hip and knee surgeries, and post stroke or to help regain prior strength and to improve gait and balance.

Physical therapy goals can include helping you move better, restoring or increasing strength and endurance, coordination, and balance.

The most common cause of falls in a nursing home is weakness and gait problems, affecting more than 80% of the residents. Nearly 3/4th of the people living in a nursing home require assistance with walking or cannot walk.

Physical therapy almost always includes exercise such as stretching, weight lifting, and walking. Your physical therapist may teach you an exercise program to continue on your own or with the assistance of a CNA.

If you think you'll need any therapy when you come to live at a nursing home (now or at a later date) check out the therapy departments and who you would most likely be working with. Many nursing homes have therapy services available right in the building.

Sources: http://www.apta.org/AboutPTs/
http://www.webmd.com/painmanagement/tc/physical-therapy-topic-overview
http://www.seniorliving.org/healthcare/physicaltherapy/

WHAT YOUR FAMILY SHOULD WATCH FOR AFTER YOU HAVE MOVED IN

Urinary tract infections

Often older people don't have the common symptoms of a urinary tract infection or aren't able to express them. **UTIs can be mistaken for early dementia or Alzheimer's because the first symptoms are confusion, agitation and hallucinations.** Certainly a need to use the toilet frequently would be a red flag. I would recommend asking the nurse to do a urine dip if these symptoms show up suddenly. A urine dip is a fast, inexpensive way to check and eliminate or find a urine infection and can be done right there at the nursing home. You can reduce the risk of UTIs by making sure briefs are changed frequently, the genital area is kept clean, using the toilet instead of using the brief or bed pan, and drinking plenty of fluids. **A urinary tract infection is the most common cause of a sudden confusion or a sudden increase in confusion in an older person.**

Links:

http://www.agingcare.com/Articles/urinarytract-infections-elderly-146026.htm
http://www.aplaceformom.com/senior-careresources

Fluids

Older people become more susceptible to dehydration for a variety of reasons. They cannot conserve water as well, don't feel as thirsty and cannot respond to temperature changes as well. The elderly often eat less or even forget to eat or drink. **Signs of dehydration** can be dark urine or decreased output, skin tenting on the back of the hand near the wrist, sudden weight loss, sunken eyes and hollow cheekbones, dry mouth and lips, urinary tract infections and constipation. A person who eats less than 50% of the meal is at higher risk for dehydration. Make sure liquids are always available, are changed regularly and offered frequently. If the resident has a hard time handling a cup or glass, check with an occupational therapist for adaptive devices, such as cups with handles or weighted cups for someone with tremors. Having liquids available and special cups does no good if the resident doesn't remember to drink. Make sure staff is encouraging the intake of liquids. Remember too, that many older people do not like ice-cold beverages and that carbonated beverages can cause gas and a feeling of being full.
See more at:

http://www.h4hinitiative.com/everyhydration/different-needs-different-lifestages/hydration-andelderly#sthash.d0FwOPuj.dpuf

Safety and Restraints

Long gone are the days where you would walk into a long-term care facility and see residents tied into wheelchairs or beds. Studies of shown that these restraints (and even things we don't think of as restraints) don't stop injury but in fact can lead to serious injury. Many elderly people have broken a hip trying to climb over bed-length side rails. So how can a nursing home keep a resident safe, as independent as possible and have a good quality of life? **There are two types of restraints, a physical restraint restricts a person's movement and they cannot easily remove it. A chemical restraint is using medication to limit movement and possibly sedate.** There are federal and state laws that strictly regulate the use of chemical restraints. I am focusing on physical restraints here.

Trying to keep residents restrain free and safe can seem conflicting at times. This is when a **multidisciplinary team and you** should be setting up a meeting. The team should include the person affected, social worker, nurses, occupational and physical therapy.

Starting with the bed, there are pads that can go under the sheet that sound an alarm if the person takes too much pressure off it. Next would be a pressure sensitive pad next to the bed. An alarm would be set off if it's stepped on. Sometimes the easy fix is just making the bed lower or adding a small grab bar.

For **someone who wanders** there are Velcro belts that can go across doorways and electronic bracelets that can go on a wrist or ankle that set off an alarm if the person tries to go out a door.

Wheelchairs can be fitted with alarmed Velcro seat belts and cushions that sound an alarm if the person stands up. This would be a good place to say that wheelchair footrests are not always in the person's best interest. If the person tries to stand up while in the wheelchair they become a trip hazard. If the person in the wheelchair cannot remember to lock the wheelchair brakes, there are self-locking brakes that can be put on.

Restraints can be simply pushing a person up to a table that they can't move away from on their own or locking wheelchair brakes so they can't move. Not making sure the resident has his/her glasses on or a working hearing aid is a type of restraint. If a person is up and **walking around independently but not safely,** there are a number of things that can be done. First would be physical and occupational therapy for strengthening, balance and safer ways to do things like using the toilet or dressing. Trying canes and walkers might be an option and they do make walkers that have seats on them so a person can sit and rest when they need to. Undergarments that are padded at the hips to reduce hip fractures and well-fitting shoes can help. If the person complains of being dizzy, side effects from drugs should be ruled out as well as vertigo. Depending on the type of vertigo, you may be able to be treated by the physical or occupational therapist.

I know it's a scary thing to see someone you love being at risk of getting hurt but remember this; **the risks with restraints include falls, strangulation, loss of muscle, skin breakdown, decreased mobility, agitation, reduced bone mass, loss of dignity, increased hospital stay, increased deaths rate, incontinence and constipation. The risks without restraints is falls.**

Sources:

http://www.aafp.org/afp/2009/0215/p254.html

Falls

Falls are the leading cause of death and reduced quality of life for people over 65. There are myriad reasons for nursing home falls but weakness and gait problems combined with dizziness and confusion are the most common cause. Medications and environmental hazards that can range from wet floors to incorrect bed height also contribute to falls. **It is important to find out why the resident fell and address any conditions** that may have contributed to the fall. The resident should have any medical conditions treated, the environment should be assessed to see if grab bars, lowering the bed and so forth would make the person safer. Undergarments that have built-in hip pads can help reduce hip fracture and exercise programs under the supervision of physical and occupational therapy can improve balance, transfers and walking. Nursing homes should have **a fall prevention program** that assesses you when you first become a resident. This assessment should let them know if you are a fall risk and to do any modifications to make you safer. One fall may have been an unfortunate accident, more than one fall should include a consult with the occupational or physical therapy department for a fall assessment.

Link:
http://www.cdc.gov/HomeandRecreationalSafety/Falls/nursing.html

Vitamin D and the Elderly

Older adults are at risk for vitamin D deficiency due to a decrease in outdoor activity, changes in their diet and the ability to produce it. There is correlation between vitamin D deficiency and **increased falls, osteoporosis and fractures**. In adults, vitamin D deficiency can lead to osteomalacia (softening bones, more likely to bow and fracture), resulting in weak bones. Symptoms of bone pain and muscle weakness can indicate inadequate vitamin D levels.
Read more about vitamin D deficiency here:
http://www.medscape.com/viewarticle/500874_4

Medication

Aging generally means more health problems and more medications; your body changes can increase the possibility of side effects from medication. Ask if any medication you are on has side effects and what they are. If you start taking a medication and experience problems swallowing, dizziness, memory problems, drowsiness, confusion constipated or have diarrhea, blurry vision, rash, dry mouth, or nausea or hallucinations let your medication nurse know immediately. **It's not just prescription drugs that can cause side effects**. Antihistamines can cause confusion, constipation and delirium in the elderly. Aspirin, ibuprofen, naproxen increases potential for bleeding. Get more information here:
http://www.pfizer.com/files/health/medicine_safety/4-6_Med_Safety_for_Elderly.pdf
http://www.aarp.org/health/drugssupplements/info-07-2011/medications-olderadults-should-use-with-caution.html

Pain

Chronic pain is a major problem in the elderly population. **Most elderly people have significant pain that isn't treated or is undertreated**. Studies have shown that 66% of nursing home residents had chronic pain but 34% of the time it was not detected. Assessing pain can be complicated because of depression, denial and poor memory. Some older people believe that pain is just a part of aging. Crying, groaning, changes in walking or posture and agitated behavior can all indicate pain. If a resident has had a recent fall and exhibits any of these after the fall, a physician should be consulted.
Sources:
http://www.ncbi.nlm.nih.gov/pmc/articles/PMC3096211/
http://www.partnersagainstpain.com/paincaregiver/elderly.aspx

Depression

For some reason we tend to think of long-term care facilities as depressing but don't think of our elderly as being depressed. Unfortunately this mind-set causes older adults in nursing homes not to be diagnosed. In reality, **20 to 35% of the elderly in long-term care have some sort of depression and less than 50% those were recognized and treated**. Physical changes as we age, pain, loss of loved ones and loss of independence all can contribute to depression.

It is harder to diagnose in older people because they are less likely to say they are sad or have crying spells. More often a senior will have a change in their eating habits, complain of being tired or not sleeping well. Remember, depression is not a normal part of aging and should be treated.

Sources:

https://www.amda.com/tools/clinical/depression/De pressioninLongTermCare.pdf

http://www.agingcare.com/Articles/nursing-homedepression-147347.htm

End of Life Care, Comfort Care, Palliative Care & Hospice

We are all mortal and we will all have to face death in our own way but that doesn't mean those caring for us, on this final journey, can't make the road easier. However, the terminology can be confusing and knowing what to ask for difficult. Many are referred to late to get the most benefit from these programs. Have a conversation with your family and medical provider about what you want and what your concerns are while you are still healthy enough to do so.

End of life care

There is no exact definition of what is end of life or what end-of-life care is but it can include years. End of life care generally is defined as helping those with an incurable illness to live as well as possible until they die. The three generally accepted ways to do this are palliative care, comfort care and hospice.

Palliative care

To improve the quality of life of those with a serious disease by preventing or treating the symptoms, side effects caused by treatment, and psychological, social, and spiritual problems related to a disease or its treatment. Palliative care can include life prolonging care and would not necessarily be end of life care.

Comfort care

This would essentially be palliative care without life prolonging care. There should be a 'Do Not Resuscitate' (DNR) order in place and a DNR sticker on the outside of the medical chart. A DNR is a legal form so you don't get CPR or cardiac life support if your heart stops or you quite breathing. You have the right to change your mind and ask for CPR.

Hospice

The goal of hospice is to help you die with dignity by giving medical, psychological and spiritual support. Hospice gives palliative and comfort care along with support from staff and volunteers. You can receive hospice through Medicare if your doctor thinks you have less than 6 months to live. If you live longer than 6 months under hospice care a doctor can continue to certify that you are close to dying and Medicare can continue to pay for hospice services. If you have a recovery, you will be removed from hospice but can go back on at a later date. Sources:
http://www.nhpco.org/about/hospice-care
http://www.clevelandclinicmeded.com/medicalpub
s/diseasemanagement/hematologyoncology/palliati
ve-medicine
 http://kindethics.com/2009/06/what-is-
thedifference-between-palliative-care-comfort-
careand-hospice
http://www.nia.nih.gov/health/publication/end-
lifehelping-comfort-and-care/finding-care-end-life

ADDENDUM (the details that can get lost)

Managing your money or valuables in a nursing home

It is not recommended that you keep any substantial amount of money or good jewelry in your room. The nursing home should have a safe deposit box and keep a signed list of what is deposited. Having a few dollars and some change in your room may be a good idea if you like to go to the vending machine for a snack but having a large amount of money or jewelry that can be easily stolen is not. A person with dementia may not recognize the value of an item and may misplace it. Nursing homes will not want to be responsible for the loss or theft of money or items.

Church and Spirituality

To many seniors church is an important part of their lives. Even if the nursing home is not a church based facility, the nursing home should provide some sort of church service on Sunday. Often the local churches take turns having the Sunday service and many churches have outreach programs. If church or Bible studies are important to you don't hesitate to call the church of your choice or your current church and let them know you are going to be living at a long term facility and would like to know what they offer for nursing home ministry.

Power Wheelchairs

Motorized wheelchairs are becoming more common in long term setting. If you own a power wheelchair before you enter the nursing home you can request to take it with you but the nursing home can have a 'no power wheelchair' policy. A power wheelchair can make it easier for you to get around and be more independent but because there could be potential problems, the nursing home will probably request certain things be met before they allow you to use it. First, it is your chair, therefore you, not the home, would be responsible for repairs. Because of safety risks to yourself and other residents they will want the chair to be checked for safety and your driving skills be checked. They may have a facility policy on power wheelchairs and have you sign an agreement on how it will be used. Having a power wheelchair is a privilege, not a right.

Reminiscence/Memory box or book

A box or book containing the life story of someone with dementia, to help them remember and communicate. Photos and words gives visual reminders that can help the person feel more secure and helps word finding for communication. It helps the staff know more about the person so they can better communicate, understand and help manage the person with dementia. It also provides topics of conversation for friends and family.

To make a memory box find photos or objects that will have a meaningful memory for the person. You would first choose a topic they enjoyed, such as fishing or sewing. Find photos of the person or other family/friends engaged in the activity. Use a tackle box to add fishing lures, fish line; to a sewing box add thread, material etc. Whatever would fit in the category you choose. A shoe box that is decorated would work fine to store memories.

A memory book would be similar to a memory box because you would choose a topic(s). After you choose the topic, you would want to one or two photo for that topic. Keep the pages simple and avoid decorations that can be distracting. Each page should have a simple caption in the first person i.e. 'my mother'. Make sure the print is large enough for the person to see. Your book can have as many topics as the person can handle. As dementia progresses pages can be removed so the book is easier to handle. Place each page in a protective sleeve and make copies in case the original gets damaged or lost. Depending on the person's dementia, they may enjoy helping make the book. If a loved one is deceased having a photograph that says, 'This is my husband Paul' may be enough. For others having a photograph with a picture of the grave that says, 'My husband Paul died in 2005' may help. You will have to use your judgment when deciding what will work best. Talk to your family and staff to get a feel on what to do.

A memory box or book will help bring back good memories while helping younger family members learn about family history.

Links:

http://www.alzheimers.net/2014-02-06/memoryboxes-for-patients/

http://www.helpforalzheimersfamilies.com/alzheimers-dementia-dealing/ capturing-memories/memory-box/

Long-term care ombudsmen

Every state is required to have an Ombudsman Program to address the following issues:

Violation of residents' rights or dignity

Physical, verbal or mental abuse, deprivation of services necessary to maintain residents' physical and mental health, or unreasonable confinement

Poor quality of care, including inadequate personal hygiene and slow response to requests for assistance

Improper transfer or discharge of patient

Inappropriate use of chemical or physical restraints

Any resident concern about quality of care or quality of life

For more information go to:

http://www.ltcombudsman.org/aboutombudsmen#Ombudsman

CHECK LISTS

QUESTIONS TO ASK BEFORE YOU MOVE IN

Roommates

Available room location

Is the room attractive and how is it set up?

Staff interaction with residents

What can you bring from home (chair, television etc.?)

Telephone, television and internet connection/cost

Visitors (including pets) and areas set aside for visiting/socializing

Clothing, clothing identification, and storage of out of season clothing and personal items On site beauty shop?

Shower or bath and how often?

How are potential problems with roommates handled?

Diet, dining times, availability of water and liquids

Alcoholic beverages

Who will be your doctor in the facility?

Are the Social workers helpful?

Who is authorized to see your medical record and who can get information about you and your health?

Is the Activity Department active?

Is there a therapy department in the building offering Speech/language, Occupational and Physical therapy?

Are people being restrained or looking as if they are over medicated?

Can you bring a motorized wheelchair if you have one?

How does the facility handle end of life? Do they have a special room set aside or can they make arrangements for a room change to allow privacy. Do they do comfort care, palliative care or arrange for hospice care to come to the nursing home?

WHAT FAMILY SHOULD WATCH FOR

Changes in mood or behavior.

Bruises

Falls

Signs of dehydration

Signs of depression

Signs of over-medication or physical/mental changes after receiving medications

Sudden weight gain or loss/too much weight gain or loss

Any restraints including medication, foot rests that prevent you from moving yourself, being left for long periods in front of a window or television, being pushed up to a table that you can't back away from, being left in bed beyond what is reasonable. Call buttons are where you can reach them. Safety alarms are in place and other safety measures are being followed.

Pain, and that it is taken seriously and being treated.

Missing money, jewelry or clothing.

Are hearing aids and teeth in, glasses on?